I0487233

HEY MEN, LISTEN UP!

HOW TO GET IT UP AND KEEP GETTING IT UP

A self help book on erectile dysfunction
Fletcher C. Derrick Jr., MD, Urologist

ISBN: 1439264759

ISBN-13: 9781439264751

PROLOGUE

This "manual" is written to help men keep and/or restore their sexual and erectile function. It is written to show men how they can help themselves when the realization of poor erectile function occurs. When the self-help is not working, then I will tell them how to get to the doctor of their choice and what may be available to help with the problem.

This booklet is not written as a scientific treatise. With few exceptions, the content is entirely from my own urological experience and practice, which began in 1960.

ABOUT THE COVER

The cover was designed by the author. When he and his wife visited Karnak Temple near Luxor, Egypt, Dr. Derrick thought the 134 columns represented a marvelous collection of phallic symbols. The temple has been there since about 1351bc. Many photos were taken and filed away for future use in lectures and teaching. This book actually had its genesis at that time. When the book was completed, the photos were found and converted to digital images so that the best could be placed on the cover.

CHAPTER 1
What is Erectile Dysfunction?

Definition: At some point the word *impotence* was replaced with the all inclusive term, *erectile dysfunction* (ED). The former word implies inability to achieve a penile erection for sexual intercourse; the new, current term includes any underlying cause creating an erectile problem. ED can occur because of a psychological problem (e.g., anxiety/depression, etc.) or because of a physical or organic problem (e.g., diabetes/hypertension, etc.). I will use the ED abbreviation from this point on, unless the text requires a better term or explanation.

Estimates from various sources reveal that 20–30 million men or more in the U.S. have ED to some degree. Some experience problems as early as their twenties and thirties. Information available from Europe and the rest of the world estimates that as many as an additional thirty million men experience ED. In the early age group (twenty to forty), most ED problems are related to psychogenic problems, e.g., stress, performance anxiety, loss of attraction, sexual hang-ups, and as I often say, money, job, children, smoking, alcohol and other drugs, in-laws, family in general, and depression. In the fifty-plus group, the problems are mostly related to organic problems (diseases that begin to show up, e.g., hypertension, diabetes, heart trouble, and peripheral vascular disease, etc.).

If you are reading this booklet, have ED, and are around forty years of age, then you have a head start. If you are fifty, you may have a little catching up to do. If you are in the sixty to seventy age group, you are behind, but there is hope. You need to listen, read carefully, and slowly work your way back into good function. It is very important to realize that ED may be the direct result of one or more of the above mentioned problems. But more importantly, it may also be the first indication of rather insidious or silent onset of hypertension, diabetes, elevated cholesterol, or other medical and hormonal problems.

CHAPTER 2
When Does Erectile Dysfunction Occur?

Erectile function is so natural from ages thirteen to fourteen until about forty to forty-five, men think it will just be that way forever. However, through weight gain, alcohol consumption, workaholism, stress, disease, etc., changes occur ever so slowly. Our bodies are quite adept at compensating, but there is a limit to this compensation. Sooner or later—and sooner in a lot of cases—the body has trouble compensating, and various systems begin to show signs of failure. Lack of physical conditioning and less-than-nutritious eating lead to: excessive weight gain, diabetes, hypertension, arteriosclerosis (hardening of the arteries), and many other problems.

This manual is primarily for the guys with physical problems. We will address men's health and erectile and sexual function, but won't get into psychology in depth. Psychosexual physicians and practitioners have covered this side of ED quite well and continue to comment on a regular basis in just about every type of broadcast and written outlets. The old adage, "It's all in your head," is quite true, but as one ages, other factors enter the equation. My favorite statement to patients is: "One still needs to be in the right frame of mind and have a willing, if not eager partner." (I have never completely understood how a man can perform sexual rape, that is, get and keep an erection while the female is under severe duress.) It takes "two to tango"; as the Ray Charles song says: "Two to get the feeling of romance, two to do the dance of love." I firmly believe this.

Unfortunately, we are a pill society. If it hurts, take a pain pill; if I'm down, take an upper; if I'm up, take a downer. If I am overweight, take a diet pill and still eat all I want. We want it all, and now. Someone was once heard praying: "Good Lord give me patience, and I want it right now!" However, pills may not always work, and getting results may take a little or a lot of effort on your part and that of your partner.

"Erectile dysfunction is a portal into men's health," said one study's senior author Aksam Yassin, from the Segeberger Clinic in Germany. "It is becoming clear that obesity, diabetes, high blood pressure, cholesterol problems and erectile difficulties are intertwined, and a common denominator is testosterone deficiency." For some men, ED is the first sign of other physical troubles. Once in a while, any man may experience an occasional episode of ED. However, at any age, if this continues, I highly suggest that one seek medical attention in that ED may be the fore runner of other medical problems.

CHAPTER 3
What Can I Do On My Own?

JUST REVIEW YOUR LIFE AND LIFESTYLE AND SEE IF SOME CHANGES ARE NOT IN ORDER.

Take a look at weight gain, smoking, alcohol, and heavy work load combination.

- If one comes home from a twelve-hour work day, eats a big meal, and has a few drinks, it's no wonder performance begins to fade.

- Take time to work out the schedules of the children and work.

- Cutting back on some of the PTA, hunting and fishing, golf, church, hobbies, and other activities can make a big difference.

- There are several "lifestyle changes" that may make a big difference. I encourage men to make these changes, but with the idea that it will be a lifelong process of keeping their body functioning at its very, very best. Having said that, I am fully aware of aging, but the data is in and accumulating every day. We can't turn the clock backwards, but we can slow aging and keep our bodies working on into the seventies and eighties. It just takes some work and help from a urologist or like physician who can recommend medications, appliances, or surgery.

• Talk to your partner. Possibly there is some very minute problem that is creating anxiety and preventing you from getting and keeping a good erection. There may be some hang-up that is working on your mind. I often say it is the diversion that interrupts the plan, such as the phone or door bell ringing, or a mental image that interrupts the game. Men generally are not talkers. They say, "Ah, nothing is wrong," and they just keep on going, only to learn in the future that the "old boy" is just not working as it has in the past. Men, it is very macho to sit down and hash it out with your spouse. Often, a light comes on when one of the other says, "Oh! I didn't know that bothered you." The revelations that come from a good talk lead to some very wonderful intimate moments. Also, you not only find out what may be a bother, but you also share ideas about what turns you on. This raises the passion level. It's okay to ask your partner to touch you in the most sensitive areas of your body. My most revered professor said in one of his lectures, "Whatever goes on between and man and his wife in the bedroom is okay." One of my patients said he was glad he married a teacher. She required that they do it over, and over, and over until they got it right—and they were still working on it, after decades of happy married life.

THE INTIMACY OF SEXUAL INTERCOURSE BETWEEN COUPLES IS A LEARNING EXPERIENCE

After we start our treatment, one of the first things I tell my older patients is that the best idea is to "make a date." The days of jumping in the bed, have a little touchy-feely, and making out are just about gone. If you make a date, then everyone is on the same page and this gives one something to think about and get prepared. Take the "pill" an hour or so ahead, take a shower, etc. (more about this later).

One deterrent to sex is when a family member moves back in, be it a child that has come home after college, or an older parent or relative. One of my patients told me that an older family member had moved into the bedroom next to the master bedroom. Each time they tried to have sex, the wife would say, "Sh! Don't want to wake Grandma!" or "Don't want to let Grandma know that we are having sex at our age."

There are several remedies. Make a date for Grandma and get her out of the house for the weekend. Or better, go away for a few days on business and/or pleasure and go to a hotel/motel. There is always something naughty about having your lover by your side and placing the key in the lock or slot of a motel. When the light turns green and the door opens, that is a nice feeling. No interruptions, no hurry, completely relaxed.

Many of my patients have told me that they have no sexual trouble away from home.

Work on your nutrition/diet plan.

• There is ample evidence in both the scientific and lay literature that a high protein, low carbohydrate nutrition plan works and has no deleterious effect on the body. Atkins diet and South Beach diet lean this way—no pun intended.

• For years, I have been telling patients to adhere to this simple diet plan:

First, white meat, colored vegetables, nuts, eggs, lean pork or beef filet, and no sugar (or as little as possible). Sugar is probably the worst culprit or the main culprit in obesity, insulin-resistant diabetes, hypertension, hardening of arteries, and other cardiac problems. Pure sugar or starch causes an outpouring of insulin. Insulin's job is to take glucose and put it into a fat cell to clear the blood of sugar and starch. It's easy to put that sugar in a fat cell, but hard to get it out. The nutrition plan that we recommend is high protein and low-glycemic-index carbohydrates, and it really seems to work. This plan, according to Dr. Barry

Sears, keeps us "in the zone" with minimal highs and lows of rapidly changing blood sugars. In my opinion, the book *Enter the Zone* by Dr. Barry Sears should be required reading for diabetics.

Go to www.nutricoach.net for a great chart on various foods and their glycemic index.

Next in the nutrition plan is counting calories: 3500 calories is a pound, coming or going. I suggest you get a calorie counter (available in most all book stores) and become familiar with the number of calories in your favorite foods.

Go to www.thecaloriecounter.com and get just about all the information you need on calories.

In the final analysis, most adult men who will get on a 1500- to 1800-calorie-per-day diet plan will lose weight and not be hungry. And, they will begin to reverse some of the effects of a high carbohydrate and sugar diet.

In history, Genghis Khan and the Mongols were the greatest conquerors. The Mongol soldier had a high-protein diet, mostly dried or fresh animal flesh and milk and milk products. They could go for days and days on those small portions of high protein. The Western European had a high-grain, high-bread diet, and they were soon famished with the low blood sugar that follows a few hours after a high carbohydrate meal. Mongols had beef jerky equivalent. They had none of the low blood sugar crashes exemplified by the after meal "downer" (*Genghis Khan and the Making of the Modern World*, Jack Weatherford, Three Rivers Press, New York 2004).

CHAPTER 4
Do Drugs and Alcohol Have an Impact on Erectile Dysfunction?

Cut back on alcohol consumption and/or recreational drugs.

All of the recreational drugs release inhibitions but interfere with performance by either interfering with the circulation or lowering testosterone.

• Ethanol: Although small amounts of alcohol may increase sexual desire by lowering inhibitions, it does not necessarily increase sexual arousal. Even in small doses, ethanol causes men's erections to be less firm. The twenty-one–year-old college student usually does not experience this after a frat party, but time will take its toll.

• "In men, alcohol causes impotence through several mechanisms. Long-term use of alcohol reduces testosterone levels and increases estrogen levels, which can result in impotence. Short-term use can cause transient impotence through alcohol's sedative effect. Additionally, alcohol can affect the nerves of the penis, causing neurogenic impotence."

• "Hormonal changes caused by long-term alcohol use can cause reduction in libido, in addition to causing impotence. Using alcohol in combination with other depressants can amplify this effect" (IsHak 58).

• Marijuana: "Long-term use of marijuana generally has a negative effect on sexuality. Chronic heavy use of marijuana can lower libido. There is some evidence that it can cause psychogenic erectile dysfunction as well" (IsHak 58). "Long-term use of marijuana can lower sperm production or cause sperm to develop abnormally. It can also lower testosterone levels. Both of these effects go away after marijuana use ceases" (IsHak 59).

• Cocaine: "As with all of the stimulants, cocaine can cause erectile dysfunction but in moderate doses, the effect of neurogenic contraction of penile trabecular smooth muscle may lead to priapism. Men generally find it very difficult to ejaculate on high doses of cocaine." "Chronic heavy use of cocaine can lower the libido" (IsHak 59).

• "Amphetamine-like drugs can increase one's desire for sex, but often makes achieving and maintaining an erection difficult. Conversely, in moderate doses, amphetamine may occasionally cause priapism. Male amphetamine users also report penile 'shrinkage'" (IsHak 60).

• Opioids, i.e., heroin, morphine, Demerol, Oxy and Hydro Condone: "Opioids can reduce sexual responses in both sexes. Men on opiates have difficulty achieving erections and ejaculating, while women on heroin produce less vaginal lubrication and have more difficulty reaching orgasm. Heavy use of opiates can lower the libido" (IsHak 61). Men taking opioid analgesics (such as Vicodin, OxyContin, or Lortab, etc.) for more than a month to relieve chronic pain can experience hormonal disturbances leading to sexual dysfunction, reports the Pain Treatment Topics website. Author Stephen Colameco notes that chronic pain and sexual problems often go together. However, doctors rarely ask about patients' sexual concerns, and guidance literature on the subject is relatively scarce.

• Amyl Nitrate and Butyl Nitrate (poppers): "Poppers are often used as sexual enhancers. They release nitric oxide, causing erection and relaxation of the rectum, facilitating anal sex. Although they can be legally purchased, poppers can increase the risk of heart failure" (IsHak 61).

• Stop smoking. Nicotine: "Nicotine can affect erectile tissue and the muscles involved in producing an erection, thus causing impotence. Men who smoke tobacco are twice as likely to be impotent as non-smoking men of the same age. Using nicotine in combination with cardiac drugs, antihypertensive medications or vasodilators drastically increases the probability of complete impotence" (IsHak 61).

CHAPTER 5
What Kind of Exercise Program Do We Recommend?

Work out an exercise program.

What kind of program? Results of a study reveal that exercise can help preserve DNA and slow the aging process. Exercise also helps to reduce stress. In an article by Dr. Bob Delmontique, he recommends doing at least twenty minutes of exercise per exercise session, five times per week. That's only 100 minutes total each week. Choose a form of exercise that you enjoy doing or a combination. Examples: brisk walking, bicycling, swimming, hiking, aerobics, or calisthenics. Delmontique also provides a table with example exercise plans to reach the 100 minutes per week goal (Delmonteque, Bob, N.D. "Slow the Hands of Time with Exercise," *Journal of Longevity.* Vol. 14/ No. 3. 2008, pages 11–12).

There are many choices: jogging, walking, biking, swimming, gym work outs, hiking, etc.—just as long and you do it.

I have heard it all: "My knees keep me from jogging," "My back keeps me from hiking," "My feet keep me from walking," etc. Some people just don't like to exercise. However, if one is to keep in reasonably good physical condition, keep their weight stable, or lose a few pounds, it is sure easier and necessary to burn a few more calories than one consumes.

If riding a street bike or stationary bike is your choice of exercise, remember that prolonged pressure on the crotch can damage the nerves and arteries that go to the penis. Choose a gel seat or one that is ergonomically designed to minimize this pressure. Most avid cyclist know about this, but I still have an occasional patient who did not get the word and comes in with some erectile dysfunction and states that his penis gets numb sometimes after a long bike ride.

Power Plate is a vibration machine (whole body vibration) that came out of the Russian space program as they were searching for methods of preserving the bone and muscle of their cosmonauts in zero-gravity of space. Data is increasing that use of the machine will build bone strength, decrease joint pain, help in loss of belly fat, and result in some improvement in neurological diseases such as Parkinson's. I have no experience with the machine and simply refer you to us.powerplate. com or **www.orthometrix.net** for more information. More information may be available at drdavidwilliams.com and his newsletter *Alternatives*, Volume 12, No. 17, November 2008.

On any given day one may read pro and con messages about supplements. I have taken the position that most don't harm and some may do good.

• Vitamins and supplements: Much is written about vitamins and food supplements. The claims made in ads and direct mail would have one believe that all of them work all of the time. Well, some of them may work part of the time.

• Most physicians say if you are getting a well balanced diet, the need for vitamins and supplements is far less than if you are eating a lot of fast food. However with depletion of soils, the nutritional content of our veggies may be low. Consuming "organic" foods may help.

• Certainly, a good "One A Day" vitamin will not hurt and may be of some help. There is more and more evidence that the antioxidants will make a great difference in our health and aging. Vitamins A, C, E, zinc, selinium, phytochemicals in vegetables, and lycopenes in tomatoes, etc., have been shown to be very necessary and beneficial. There is also extremely good evidence that fish oil and flax oil (DHA) is great for general health.

CHAPTER 6
What About The Drugs and Medications Seen in Advertisements

"What about the drugs and medications for ED in advertisements?"

Almost daily we see ads in newspapers, magazines, and special mailings informing us of the "most potent sexual enhancer ever." Scores of testimonials are enclosed that speak of the greatness of the product. As a urologist for over forty-nine years, I can report that most of these products do not work as well as advertised. Most don't work at all. Yes, there is the placebo effect in some men, but these are few and far between. The ingredients do have some properties that may enhance erectile performance, but there is always the chance of having an untoward reaction to these products. The following are the most common ingredients in these supplements.

• Pygeum africanum: The bark from this tree has been used "to treat bladder and urination disorders, particularly symptoms associated with benign prostatic hypertrophy (BPH), which is an enlarged prostate." It has been "observed to moderately improve urinary symptoms associated with enlargement of the prostate gland or prostate inflammation" (Medline).

• Bromelain: An herb from the pineapple plant. It is believed that Bromelain can help in protein digestion and also as an anti-inflammatory agent. Some believe it helps those suffering from Peyronie's disease. Enteric-coated Bromlain is now being touted for arthritis (Medline).

• Saw palmetto: The most popular herbal treatment for benign prostatic hypertrophy (BPH), enlargement of the prostate. Uses are based on tradition or theory: hormone imbalances, impotence, sexual vigor, testicular atrophy, sperm production. (Medline). It may provide modest relief of urinary symptoms. Long-term safety and effectiveness are not known. The federal government does not oversee dose, quality, or purity. Side effects include occasional mild stomach upset and diarrhea (*The Post and Courier*, 2D, Monday, August 4, 2008, Harvard Medical School Advisor).

Supplements that seem to enhance effects of nitric oxide (the potent vasodilator necessary for erection):

• L-Arginine: This amino acid is the body's natural precursor to nitric oxide, which is the potent vasodilator necessary for erection. I have recommended L-Arginine to many men who find that it is quite helpful. It is being used not only for erectile dysfunction but some practitioners are recommending L-Arginine for treatment of hypertension. They are getting the vasodilation effect of L-Arginine. It is available without prescription and has shown some good results in treating ED. It has been called "the poor man's Viagra." Capsules of 500 mg can be taken twice daily.

• Watermelons: Recently, watermelons were cited as being a good aphrodisiac for men because they contain a high content of citrulline, which is changed to L-Arginine, which is subsequently changed to nitric oxide. Now, citrulline is available as a food supplement.

• DHEA: "Dehydroepiandrosterone" produced in the adrenal glands diminishes in the aging male. Men who have only moderate changes in their libido or moderately low serum testosterone may benefit from DHEA, which is available without prescription. It has actually been touted by some experts as being the anti-aging hormone. The dose is 25–50 mg daily. There seems to be minimal-to-no side effects. The same precautions about prostatic specific antigen should be taken—be sure your physician checks your PSA when taking DHEA.

• Yohimbine hydrochloride: A prescription drug that has been shown in multiple human trials to effectively treat male impotence. Yohimbine may also be a useful treatment option in orgasmic dysfunction. Yohimbine, yocon, thybine, afrodyne, etc., are parasympathetic nervous system stimulators that seem to work about 50% of the time in improving sexual activity. I always tell my patients that yohimbine will not increase sex drive. It helps one perform better once foreplay has started and may assist in those with delayed ejaculation or with the loss of erection during intercourse. Yohimbine has helped many men with ED just due to aging process (men who don't have diabetes, hypogonadism, or hypothyroidism).

For some products advertised regularly and their ingredients, I simply suggest that you be very careful in using any of these products for the reasons mentioned above. They all may have some value, but most use the same or nearly the same ingredients, which may or may not be helpful. I particularly suggest that older patients who are already taking heart, blood pressure, or diabetic and other medications be very careful in taking these supplements.

• Enzyte: contains Korean gensing and ginko biloba, horny goat weed extract, L-arginine, tribulus terrestris extract, avena sativa extract, pine bark extract, maca root, puama extract (aerial part), saw palmetto berry, swedish flower pollen extract, niacin, zinc, copper.

• Vicerex: contains tongkat ali, Malaysian gensing long jack, horny goat weed, tribulus terrestris, maca (powerful Peruvian aphrodiasiac), gingko biloba, ying yang huo (Chinese herb).

• ViSwiss: contains yohimbine bark, epimedium, ashwaganda root (Indian gensing), avena sativa, gingko biloba, Korean gensing, Peruvian gensing, muira puama (Brazilian tree root and bark), saw palmetto, tribulis terrestris.

• VigRxPlus: with bioperine, clinically proven to increase herbal absorption rates. Contains most of the other herbs of the other products plus damiana, epimedium leaf extract, cuscuta seed extract, cutauba bank extract.

• ExtenZe: This one is supposed to enhance the size of the penis. No real new ingredients that I could determine. Be careful, because their website will place you on auto order, and you have to call or email to stop—sometimes this can be trouble.

The FDA has identified several of these products which may contain potentially harmful, undeclared ingredients. Some of them listed on a FDA Site are: Actra-Rx, HS Joy of Love, Actra-Sx, Libidus, Vigor-25, 4ERERON, Energy Max, Natural-Up, Blue Steel, Erextra, Super Shangai, Hero, and Adam Free.

CHAPTER 7
MALE SIZE ENHANCEMENT DEVICES

- ProExtender (Penis Traction Device)

- Size Genetics (Penis Extender Review)

I have looked at many of these products and had many discussions with other urologists and there is really *no way* to enlarge the penis. There may be a few exceptions, but very, very few. The vacuum erection devices will be discussed later. They will help with erection, but do nothing for size enhancement.

SURGERY TO INCREASE PENILE SIZE

There is *no way* to increase penile size. Some surgeons have released the suspensory ligament at the pubis, which gives the appearance of more length to the flaccid penis, but not to the erect one. As a matter of fact, when the suspensory ligament is released, the erect penis does not "stand up" as it usually will. Others tout penile creams, penile stretchers, penile exercises, etc., in various advertisements. I tell the truth when I say in my experience none of these methods work in making the penis larger.

Hey Men, Listen Up!

Some surgeons have promoted injections of a person's own fat (or in some cases a special mixture of collagen) into and under the penis skin. This may give a temporary enlargement and thickness to the penis, but over time, this injection material seems to either dissipate or turn into lumps, making the appearance of the penis not smooth.

SIZE OF PENIS AND FEMALE SATISFACTION

I have seen many men who had the impression that their penis was small. Please refer to the size chart. Flaccid, the penis can seem or actually be very small, averaging 1–3 inches. Men have always jokingly said, in cold weather, it's hard to find. Erect, the average length of a penis is 4–6 inches. The thickness, width, or girth varies. Many surveys have been done, asking females if penis size makes a difference during sex. Most say it does not make a difference, except a few say there may be a slight advantage for the thick penis. The wide penis may rub the clitoral and labia region more vigorously during thrusting, imparting some additional sensual feelings to the female.

Many complaints come from the older set who say their penis is vanishing. As some men age, they gain weight. They may get the "beer gut," and the roll of fat on the lower abdomen simply hides the penis. The penis is actually still there, but can't rise above the fat. There is probably another reason: not having nocturnal erections and keeping the penis expanded part of the time. Please go to www.phallic.org/penis-size/ for charts on penile size.

Fletcher C. Derrick, Jr., M.D.

TRY HAVING SEX ON A FULL TANK OF ENERGY

Try having sex on a full tank of energy.

Early in a marriage, the sex is so spontaneous. It just happens without much work or planning. Years later, with children, jobs, schedules, etc., trying to have sex after a twelve-hour day, a few drinks, a big meal, and a nap on the sofa just doesn't work. Mornings are so much better, or when rested and having, as I call it, "a full tank of energy." Testosterone is normally highest in the morning between 7:00 and 10:00 a.m.

The suggestion I often make to my men is: "Make a date for some morning. Wake up, make the coffee, read the paper. Then take your wife coffee and the paper, and have a rendezvous."

FEMALE PROBLEMS

Dryness in female: In the aging female, it is possible to be very dry even with great sexual excitement. There are several substitutes: Replens and Liquid KY Jelly are two that seem to have good reports from the users.

CHAPTER 8
It's Time For A Visit With The Doctor

If none of the above seem to work:

- It's time for a visit with the doctor.

- Go alone, or go with your partner? It's probably best to go with your partner.

- After the usual introductions and learning the real reason for the visit, I ask three questions:

    - Do you have any sexual desire, or is your desire down? This is known as libido.

    - Do you get any erection at all, even the so-called nocturnal erection (nighttime erection), better known in the vernacular as the "piss hard"?

    - If you get an erection, will it remain until climax, or does it sometimes go down before climax?

Hey Men, Listen Up!

After we get an answer to the three sentinel questions, we then start with a complete patient history and physical examination. Once we get answers to all these important questions and others gleaned from the general medical history, we can then proceed as needed.

The most common complaint in a man fifty-five to seventy is he will get an erection, get started with intercourse, but then lose it somewhere along the way, sometimes even after penetration. Most men describe it as, "I was having sex and almost at the climax, for some unknown reason, the impending feeling of climax decreased and the erection left. It was very difficult to get it back even with intensive foreplay or manipulation during that session." Or, "It leaves the party before the party's over."

If a man has a good sex drive (libido) and nocturnal erections, then there is a pretty good chance he has normal testosterone. If he has no sex drive, then that means that he is probably low on hormones. If he gets no erection at all, then more than likely we are dealing with a real organic problem—circulation, diabetes, etc.

After the complete history, a complete physical is done, including a prostate exam. Basic lab tests are:

1. Testosterone levels.
2. PSA (prostate specific antigen—blood test we use to help us diagnose cancer of the prostate).
3. Thyroid screen.

4. Prolactin, FSH and LH (pituitary hormones).
5. I have started to check Hba1c (reveals if too much insulin and glucose). Check on this for young guys (thirty-two to thirty-five) who shouldn't really be having a problem with ED. A positive Hba1c could point to early or impending diabetes.

CHAPTER 9
Treatment

• Depending on the patient's situation, we may begin some treatment with either Viagra, Levitra, or Cialis to see if we can give boost to sexual performance before blood tests reports.

• Some patients have already tried these drugs with their family practitioners, and they didn't work. This becomes a bigger challenge in the treatment.

• In our experience if one works, they all work. If one does not work, another may. We certainly give patients the choice of trying all three if they don't seem to be getting good results.

Timing is very important in taking Viagra, Levitra, or Cialis.

I have always told my patients to take either of the pills on an empty stomach or before a very small meal. All of the pills reach their peak levels between 1–2 hours. Plan your encounter with this in mind.

Note about Viagra: There is a blue covering on the pill that is very slow to dissolve in some men.

Hey Men, Listen Up!

Either take it 2–3 hours ahead of your sexual encounter, or bite the pill or cut it with a pill cutter so that it will take effect quickly. It has a somewhat bitter taste.

HOW DO THESE PILLS WORK?

Nitric oxide is potent vasodilator. The "FIL" drugs—tadalafil, vardenafil, and sildenafil—stop the breakdown of nitric oxide. This enhances the normal erectile chemistry.

Point of caution: We don't like to use this category of drugs in men who either are taking or may take nitroglycerine-type medications. The reason is these medications block the breakdown of nitric oxide chemically in the body so that they are getting vasodilation by virtue of the activity of the drug. This may lead to a drop in blood pressure and untoward cardiac and circulatory events.

• Viagra: Peak onset within about an hour to hour and a half, lasting about four or five hours. When the clinical testing in England was originally designed, Viagra was to be a drug for hypertension. In the course of the evaluation, the drug did not demonstrate powerful anti-hypertensive properties so the researchers announced that the study was ending and asked participants to please return the unused drug. Some men refused to bring it back—why? It was enhancing their erections. With this serendipity, the study was redesigned and the rest is history.

• Levitra: Onset within an hour to hour and a half, lasting eight to ten hours. Some of my patients who have taken all three of these drugs seem to like the medium time of activity in the body and side effects that don't seem to linger with Livetra. (This is an observation only.)

• Cialis: Peak onset within an hour to hour and a half, lasting about thirty-six hours. This trait of the drug has been used in vast marketing, implanting the idea that when the time is right, the man will be ready. In truth, there is measurable drug still circulating thirty-six hours later, but at much lower levels than within the first three to four hours. The idea, however, is certainly good. Cialis has developed a daily drug plan, using 2.5 mg and/or 5 mg daily rather than the 20 mg big dose on demand. This may be helpful in the younger set (forty-five to fifty-five), but in my opinion, the older set (sixty to eighty), for the most part, are having sexual encounters less often, say once a week or less, and simply need to take the pill when the date is set.

Side effects of all the drugs tend to be a stuffy nose, flushing of the face, heartburn, and a droopy feeling, sometimes for twelve to twenty-four hours after the medication has worn off. There seems to be fewer side effects with Levitra and Cialis than with Viagra but these can vary with the dose of either. There are other side effects, but most are only annoying. Of course, there have been those who tried to push the envelope, taking far more than a safe dose with disastrous results. Taken as prescribed or not used if certain other drugs are already being taken, is the best plan.

Hey Men, Listen Up!

Note: I am certain I will get some calls or letters from the representatives of the companies that make the above drugs. Each wishes their product to be the "best" in every category and the "least" in causing problems. I am simply telling my readers and the world that in my experience with all of the drugs, and feedback from hundreds of patients, this is what I have seen and heard.

These drugs can be used as often as one wishes: daily, weekly, or monthly. However, we do not recommend using the full dose more than once daily. There are reports of circulatory collapse and problems with overdoses.

Here, I can say that Viagra, Cialis, and Levitra seem to be very safe.

There have been reports in the scientific literature and lay press of deaths occurring in those who took the pills. Some men have told me their wives do not want them to take the tablets. Well, I have two responses: 1. The wife is very concerned about her husband's health. 2. She does not want to have sex.

As I have said previously, using the pills outside the recommended dosage and if other medications are being taken which could cause an unfavorable reaction in the body, is not good. Otherwise, they seem to work and have very few bad side effects.

Some patients have already tried these drugs on recommendation of their family practitioners, and they didn't work. ED may be a bigger challenge.

CHAPTER 10
Diseases and Conditions Directly Related to ED

Diabetes mellitus is the most common cause of erectile dysfunction.

• Sometimes I will make the diagnosis of diabetes, or the patient may have been diagnosed already by an internist. Once diagnosed, treating diabetes comes first.

• You can control diabetes, but it's an autoimmune disease; it's not going away. Or it probably won't unless you make serious changes.

• The internist or family practitioner will always help in regulating diabetes.

• High blood pressure.

• High cholesterol.

• Metabolic syndrome, abdominal obesity, blood fat disorders (high cholesterol and other fats), insulin resistance diabetes, prothrombotic state (high clotting factors in blood), proinflammatory state (high C reactive protein in blood): All these patients have an increased incidence of vascular problems such as heart attacks and strokes.

- Cardiovascular disease.

- Atherosclerosis.

- Neurological diseases (multiple sclerosis, Post CVA or stroke, diabetic neuropathy).

- Hormone disorders:

    Thyroid
    Hypogonadism (Low testosterone caused by poor pituitary or testicular function).
    Hyper-Prolactinemia, prolactin is a hormone produced in the pituitary which blocks effects of testosterone. A few men have such a pituitary tumor.

Other physical factors

- Surgery/recovery (colon, aortic aneurysm).

- Stomach ulcers and hiatal hernia.

- Medications:

    - The patient's medication list is always reviewed in course of evaluation.

    - Lipitor and all other statin drugs. These all lower testosterone to some degree. Cholesterol is a building block of testosterone.

• Urological drugs (Flomax, Uroxatral, Avodart, Proscar): Used to reduce the size of an enlarging prostate and to improve the urine flow in older men, may cause retrograde ejaculation and or decrease in libido.

• Anti-depressants retard ejaculation. (Prozac has actually been effective treatment for premature ejaculation.)

• Opiates (Percocet, Percodan, Lortab, Demerol, Oxycontin, etc.)

• Propecia (Fenesteride), used for hair loss. Same as Proscar but lower doses.

• Tagamet (anti-testosterone), used to treat ulcers.

• Nicotine.

• Recreational drugs (marijuana, heroin, cocaine, etc.).

• Alcohol.

• Barbiturates.

• Amphetamine.

• Antihistamines.

• "Cold" medications: they all usually contain antihistamines and a vasoconstrictor.

Hey Men, Listen Up!

One other problem that needs some attention

Peyronnie's Disease: A scarring or thickening (called *plaque*) of the elastic membrane of the penis. The cause is unknown, but may have something to do with prolonged penetration and rubbing on the pelvic bones of the female.

• Symptoms: A bending of the penis when erect. This can be as gentle bend that is hardly noticeable to an angulation that either prevents penetration or makes it difficult and uncomfortable for the male or female. Some men have pain in the penis. The pain can occur in a flaccid penis or only when an erection occurs. The pain can be very annoying and interfere with intercourse and erection.

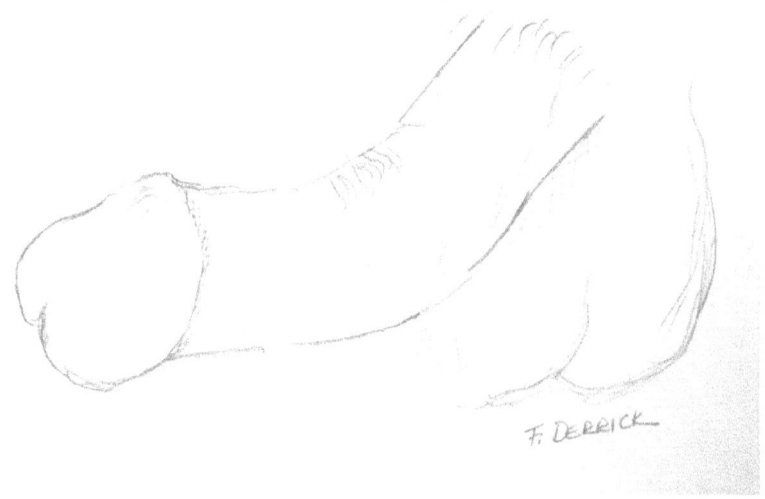

Angulation of Penis Caused by The Peyronie's Disease Scar.

- Treatment

  - Vitamin E, 400 units daily for several months. Be sure to get Alpha and/or Gamma Tocopherol, not dextro-levo.

  - A prescription medication called Potaba (para-aminobenzoate).

  - Injections of Verapamil (into the plaque or lesion), a calcium antagonist hypertensive drug.

  - Injections of cortisone (into the plaque), or with a cream rubbed on the penis and delivered with ultrasound directly to the skin of penis.

  - Low-dose irradiation has been used for pain control, but does very little to nothing in scar reduction.

  - Surgery is necessary in some cases to straighten the penis and/or remove portions of the plaque and replace it with some sort of graft.

  - Penile implant: Some men do quite well with a penile implant, which is performed in conjunction with straightening or removal of some plaque.

Hey Men, Listen Up!

Beginning treatment

- Treat lifestyle factors—improve general health.

This is where to discuss diet plan. Patients need to step up and take control of these issues when treatment for ED begins. Regardless of whether a man needs medication, hormones, etc. there are important lifestyle changes all men should adopt.

After we have done our interview and after finding through examination that nothing is out of the ordinary, I almost always will include counseling about lifestyle, weight, dietary considerations.

Then, of course, depending on lab results, if the patient has an elevated PSA, then I have to evaluate that more carefully, which may mean a repeat of the test to know whether it was high or not. Of course, that needs to be evaluated to make sure he doesn't have cancer of the prostate.

Vacuum erection devices (VED)

This is a plastic tube system in which the patient creates negative pressure, allowing the penis to inflate. A rubber band is placed at the base to allow the erection to remain for a few moments. This can be used in conjunction with Viagra, Cialis or Levitra or other medications with the precautions as mentioned previously.

Fletcher C. Derrick, Jr., M.D.

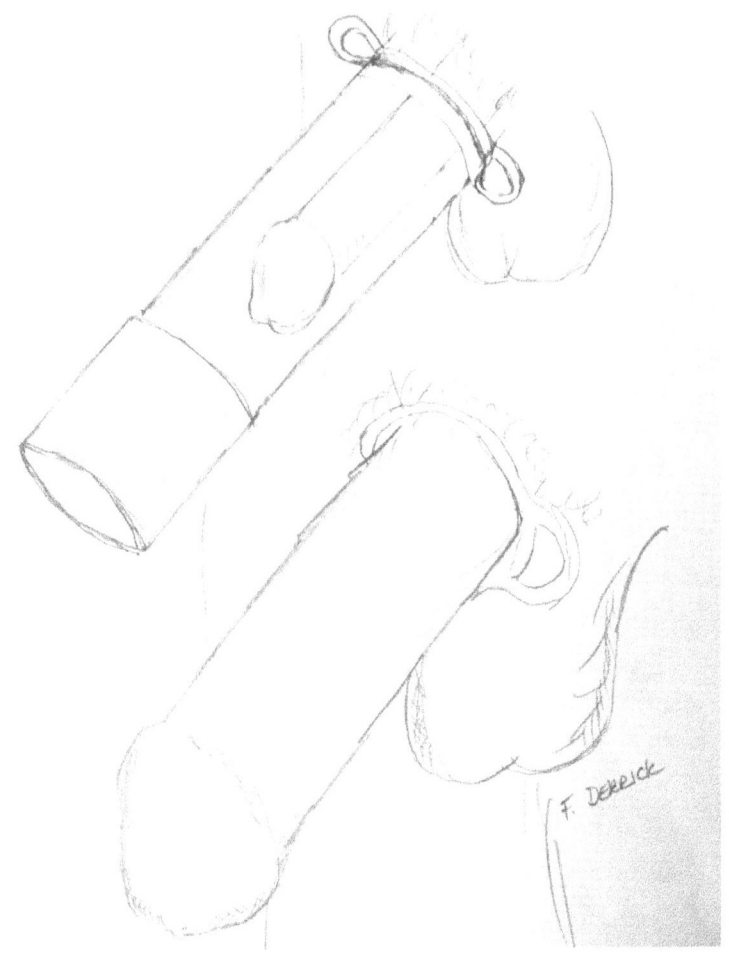

Vacuum Erection Device to Obtain Erection

The VED is completely non-invasive with a minimal risk of side effects.

It can be placed at any time during foreplay. There is no waiting period for medications to take effect.
It can be used in conjunction with or as a supplement to medication for erectile dysfunction.

43

Hey Men, Listen Up!

Actis Rubber Tourniquet: An easy release tourniquet for the penis. Available in most drug stores. Tension Rings. Commonly known as a "cock ring," some men use these rings to assist with holding an erection. They are available at Encore Tension Rings and Osbon Tension rings. There are metal rings available; however, they can cause a very snug fit creating a prolonged erection. There are reported cases of these metal rings having to be removed with metal cutters in the emergency rooms or operating rooms.

MUSE Insertion Technique

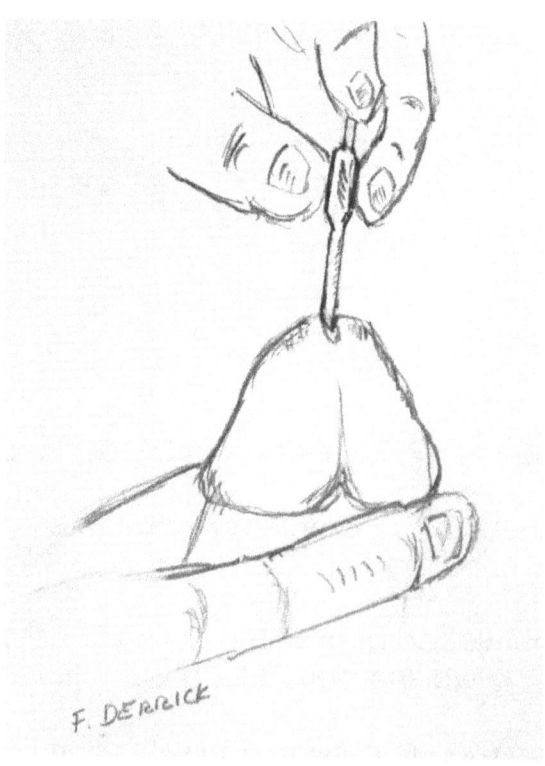

MUSE: prostaglandin urethral suppository

The MUSE Urethral Suppository comes in four dose sizes. It works well for some men. Not many men get used to the idea of inserting the pellet into the penis.

Intracorporeal (IC) Injection

In men who have had little or no response to other medications such as Viagra, etc., testosterone, thyroid, there is almost a sure guarantee of getting an erection by the IC method. We often call this "erection on demand."

Originally, Papaverine was used. However, it did create some priapism—(continuous erection over a very long period of time). Subsequently, Phentolamine was added, which enhanced the effectiveness of each drug working in tandem. But again, priapism was to some degree a problem. Then Prostaglandin E-1 was added to the mix, making what is today known commonly as "trimix." Using very small doses of each medication rather than large doses of a single medication, erection is enhanced greatly, with the length of time of the erection can be "titrated," or tailored, for the individual. The dose will be determined by your urologist, usually with a test dose first to see the effects.

The wonderful part about the IC is that it has virtually no effect on the rest of the body. I don't know of a contraindication for using trimix to assist with an erection. It works about 90–95% of time. The only minor problems with the IC are occasional bruising at the site of injection, particularly in men taking anti-coagulates (blood thinners), and occasionally a minor discomfort in the penis even though erection is gone, which probably has to do with the prostaglandin in the mix.

The trimix is a prescription product provided by your physician in his/her office or from a compounding pharmacy. In my office, we have an instruction visit and inject the first dose, giving me a chance to instruct the patient in the procedure and making sure the patient has no untoward reaction. If it works well and the patient can do it (or his partner), then we give explicit instructions by way of CD or video and written instructions. Ninety-five percent of the men who have used the trimix injection are quite pleased and continue to use it. (Yes, there are "drop outs" from this program.)

• There are two other direct injection products on the market that contain only alprostadil (Prostaglandin e-1). They are Edex and Caverject.

• Trimix gel: In December 2008, Trimix Laboratories LLC introduced a "New Generation "TriMix-gel"® is a gel that is mixed at the time of usage and inserted into the urethra. I have had no experience with this product in my patients.

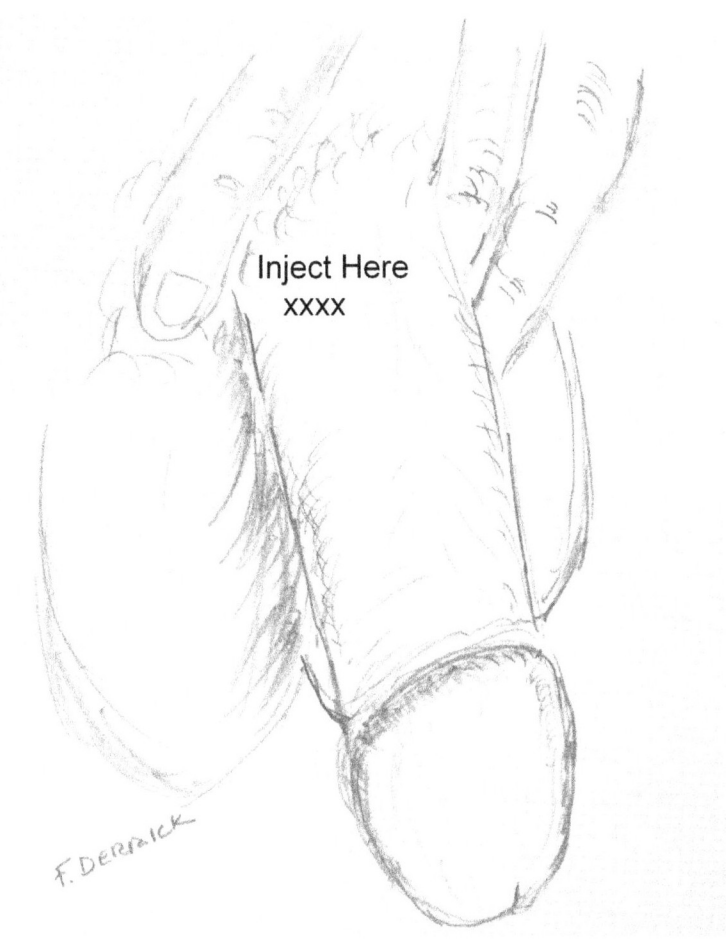

Inject Here
xxxx

F. DERRICK

A simple technique to inject the Trimix. Use the fingers of one hand to push the fat and hairs back making the penis more visible. Inject at about 2-3 o'clock or 9-10 o'clock on the penis.

Hormone Replacement Therapy

Testosterone replacement therapy depends somewhat on the patient's ability to pay.

Hey Men, Listen Up!

A prescription is necessary, and testosterone is a controlled substance.

• The oral or pill form of testosterone currently approved by the FDA in the USA simply does not work well and has some untoward side effects. There is a medication called Testosterone Undecanoate, which is an oral form of testosterone that is not approved by the FDA. It is available in Canada and most of the rest of world.

Buccal: A form of testosterone that is held in the mouth like a Tootsie Roll. The active testosterone is absorbed through the mucous membrane of the mouth. Although innovative, it has not been used by patients and doctors as often as the other types of delivery systems.

• Gel: A monthly dose of gel or patch can run about $250 if the patient has to pay out of their pocket. If insurance coverage is provided, it could be $50 depending on co-pay.

• AndroGel and Testim: Both are rubbed on in measured doses, in a hairless portion of the body—hip, shoulder, lateral/chest. It usually deliver 25–50 mg of testosterone, of which about 10–20% is absorbed. So that over the course of a month, a person will get a full dose of 300 to 400 mgs.

• Once the gel is rubbed on the body you should not swim, shower, or sweat profusely for about eight to ten hours. That's easy for some people.

• It can rub off on another person. So one must be careful holding a child, for example, and it could rub off on a sexual partner, which may not be all bad, in that testosterone drives libido in females also.

Injection
Quick, minimally painful, and very effective.

• Testosterone in oil or "depo" testosterone. The usual dose is 300–400 mgs every three to four weeks. There are variations on the doses. Frequently we teach patients to give themselves or have a family member give the injection if they have medical/health training.

• Testopel, or testosterone pellets. Pellets can be injected under the skin and last four to six months. We have just begun to use this type of testosterone replacement, but it seems to be working well. A very minor surgical procedure taking about fifteen minutes is necessary to implant the pellets. Be sure to get pre-certification for Testopel. The cost is about $800.

• After we start testosterone then we recheck in about six to eight weeks to see if we have a therapeutic level, and we also recheck the PSA.

• The dogmatic statement is, "Testosterone does not cause cancer of the prostate." But we have to be vigilant because there is an occasional case of occult (hidden) cancer that is not detected by a high PSA. All the more reason to check the PSA in a few months after starting testosterone therapy and annually. In my own private practice experience, after over forty years of using testosterone for hypogonadism, I have had only two cases out of hundreds of men who had a rising PSA while be treated for hypogonadism. They both were determined to have cancer and received appropriate treatment.

In men who have had complete removal of the prostate for prostate cancer, who either had or develop hypogonadism (low testosterone) with a PSA of 0 for four to five years, there seems to be no reason to withhold testosterone therapy.

• At the time of this writing, there is increasing evidence that men who develop cancer of the prostate actually have low testosterone. The opposite theory is that men who maintain a normal testosterone as they age or have treatment for hypogonadism may have some protection against the development of cancer of the prostate.

• Testosterone replacement in diabetic is sometimes difficult. They don't respond quite as well, and I have to check the estradiol levels—these may be at unbalanced levels and may require additional hormone replacement besides testosterone.

- DHEA: I mention this again, because it is a nice way to replace hormones in those who do not have very low testosterone but still need some support in this area. Dehydroepiandrosterone is produced in the adrenal gland and is diminished in the aging male. Some men who have only a moderate change and moderately low serum testosterone, may benefit from DHEA, which is a pill. It has actually been touted by some experts as being the anti-aging hormone. The doses about 25–50mg daily. There seems to be minimal-to-no side effects. The same precautions about PSA should be taken—double check PSA while taking.

- Replacing thyroid hormones: A certain percentage of patients will have low thyroid and will need replacement, after which there is a great possibility they will pep up with physical and sexual energy as well.

Okay, now that we know all the treatments, what do I recommend?

Trial and response

I usually give my patients a sample of the medication with instructions to call me if it works. If it does not work, we will try another.

Combination of treatments

I have number of patients who get a fair response to the "FIL" medications, but not enough to penetrate and last during the act of intercourse.

Hey Men, Listen Up!

This is when I suggest a combination therapy of pill and trimix penile injection. Some of these patients are also on testosterone.

MY ADAGE IS "DO WHATEVER IT TAKES TO WORK"

CHAPTER 11
Penile Implants

SURGERY

- If all else fails, a penile implant can be inserted.

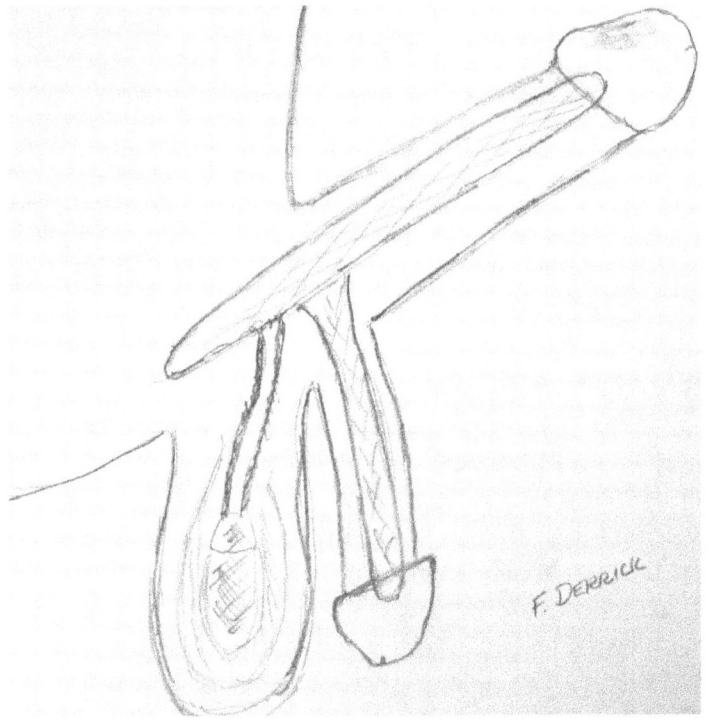

Graphic showing an inflatable penile implant in place, both in flaccid and erect position. The pump to create and release the erection is in the scrotum.

• Two types of penile implants are available: a malleable silicone rod and an inflatable balloon type implant.

• Medicare will pay for it.

• Most insurance companies who are the primary insurer of the patient will not pay for a penile implant unless the man has had prostate removal for cancer or other types of pelvic surgery such as an aneurysm or colorectal operation.

• Cost: $20,000 to $25,000 if a patient has to pay out of pocket. During my career, I have had about one patient per year who was not Medicare age who would pay for the procedure.

PREMATURE EJACULATION

Premature ejaculation has been described as ejaculation prior to penetration or ejaculation within thirty seconds of penetration. A recent study revealed that the average time from penetration to ejaculation is about 5.4 minutes. One patient, who came to me with a problem, told me of going to a strip tease show, and during the show he got an erection. When the girls finished the dance, they came to the tables asking for drinks and tips. One girl sat down beside him, asked him to buy her a drink and, in doing so, rubbed the inside of his thigh. Finding his erect penis, she laughed and said her dancing must have been very good. She got her drink and continued to rub his leg and penis, and he ejaculated in his pants. After receiving her tip, she smiled a little knowing smile and left for another customer.

Various methods have been used to help with premature ejaculation including the following:

• Use of topical Novocain or other anesthetic gels.

• Use of the "squeeze technique," which is done as follows: when the male has the feeling of impending ejaculation, he withdraws from the vagina and his partner squeezes very hard on the head of the penis with the forefinger on the opening of the urethra (the pee hole) and the thumb on the other side of the head of the penis. This actually works for some couples.

• Use of anti-depressant drugs such as Prozac. These drugs are known to retard ejaculation in those who are taking them for depression. My patients have had little success with this method.

• Psycho-sexual counseling. Some men have had good results with counseling. Some hang-up or long standing myth in their mind keeps them from holding back on the impending ejaculation.

• The other side of the argument is that some females want their partners to ejaculate quickly, because they get tired and their vaginas get sore if the thrusting goes on and on.

• General points: concern is the first time you can't do it twice, panic is the second time you can't do it once. This is about the time a man will come in for help. They may come alone or with their spouse. When I see a man or a couple less than forty to forty-five years of age, the most common problems are stress or some sort of sexual hang-up. These men do not have organic problems, they have psychological problems. Men fifty, fifty-five, sixty, and older, nearly always have organic problems, that is, high blood pressure, diabetes, etc.

A Few More Stories That Came From My Patients Which Are All True

I walked into an examine room, introduced myself to the patient, and asked the usual question: "What can I do for you?"

The patient responded, "I'm stiff in all the wrong places."

After greeting one of my eighty-year-old patients and starting our visit, I asked him, "How is your sex life?"

After looking pensive for a moment, his response was, "Quiet."

I cracked up, thinking that the opposite of quiet is noisy. I still break out laughing every time I think of it and have repeated that story hundreds of times to my other patients. My staff still wonders what the laughter coming from the exam room is all about.

One of my patients had very successful surgery for cancer of the prostate. Unfortunately, he was impotent after the procedure. After failing with medications, I offered him the trimix penile injection. He had a great response and has used it successfully for many years. After one of his checkups, I asked if he needed anything else. He quickly said, "Yes! I want some more of that rocket fuel for my heat seeking missile."

When we first started the penile implant program, patients were kept in the hospital two to three days prior to discharge. One of my patients received a get well card from a friend and couldn't wait to show it to me. It looked like the usual get well card with the words on the front, "Sorry you are sick, hope you are recovering quickly," but turning to the inside, I found the following words: "You have to stop telling the doctor to kiss it and make it well."

I had to do a cystoscopy on one of my closest friends. After he was under anesthesia, the sheet was pulled back and tucked between his penis and scrotum was one of his business cards. On the back the following message was written in his hand writing, "This had better work when you are finished." When I finished the surgery, I tucked one of my business cards in the same place with the following words, "I must be a witness to it working or not working." Needless to say we have had many a good laugh over that little incident.

Hey Men, Listen Up!

When Viagra came out, we had only the clinical trials and sales person information to give to our patients. As the patients started coming in with their responses, one of the funniest was a man who said the drug took longer than an hour to work. His taking it at eight to nine o'clock for a ten o'clock bed time just did not work. Under those conditions, it seemed to work quite well at four a.m. My comment was to tell his wife to be ready at any time. His question to me was, "How many times have you woken up your wife at four a.m. for sex?" One other patient had a similar circumstance and had this comment, "There are two things that are greatly overrated, leftover food and wakeup sex."

Another patient told me that he and his wife enjoyed sex on Sunday afternoon after church and lunch. He would place a pill in his jacket pocket and when church was over, he would go by the water fountain and take his pill. This was usually about thirty to forty minutes before lunch. When his nose began to get stuffy, he knew the medication was working. Everything worked well in the bedroom as well.

An eighty-plus-year-old patient came in and after his annual exam asked for Levitra. I approved it and added that I did not want any report of him misbehaving. He thought for a second and said, "If I misbehave, everybody is going to know it."

I have always been an advocate of and urged my men to have periodic ejaculation, at least once or twice per week, regardless of age.

I started recommending this in some of my patients with prostatitis and subsequently in all men to help keep the system working. I gave a talk to the American Academy of Family Practice in Kansas City, Missouri, once, and part of my responsibility was to make a cassette tape after the talk to be distributed to Family Practitioners by the association. It was called the Medical Minute.

Well, the tape not only went to docs, but also went to some news organizations and radio outlets. A group of my friends from South Carolina were in Alaska on a fishing trip. There was no TV in the remote camp, but there was a radio. As they were listening to the news, etc., the public service Medical Minute came on and lo and behold, it was the tape I had made in Kansas City about the ejaculation recommendation. It was greeted with great laughter, and I received a great deal of ribbing from my friends. when they returned home.. They did inform me however, that for the rest of the fishing trip, they teased each other as they went for a leak, announcing that they were going to treat their prostatitis.

A FEW WORDS ABOUT PROSTATE DISEASE

• The prostate gland is a walnut-size organ that sits at the outlet of the bladder and has one function, the production of semen. Semen is the fluid produced at ejaculation and carries the sperm into the female reproductive tract. Semen contains the nutrients and chemistry that sperm need to make the journey.

Hey Men, Listen Up!

- It is very normal for the aging male to produce less and less semen.

- It is very normal for the aging male to have some mild voiding problems, sometimes starting in the early fifties but nearly always in the seventies. Most of the symptoms are annoying and do not need treatment. However, if one is losing sleep because of the night time frequency of urination, has a slow stream, and cannot control the urination, a visit to the urologist may result in some help.

PERSONAL BIO

Dr. Fletcher C. Derrick, Jr., was born in Johnston, South Carolina, attended Johnston public schools, and earned his bachelor's in pre-med from Clemson University. He graduated from the Medical University of South Carolina in 1958. After serving his internship at Martin Army Hospital, at Fort Benning, Georgia, he and his wife Martha were stationed in Germany, first at Baumholder with the Eighth Division Artillery, and later at the 2nd General Hospital at Landstuhl, Germany.

At Landstuhl, he was given an opportunity to work in the urology wards under Dr. Prince Beach, Dr. James Fawcett, and Dr. Paul Boetger. This led to a urology residency at MUSC under Dr. Kenneth Lynch with completion in 1966. He stayed on the faculty of MUSC until 1970 when he became the professor and chairman of the department of urology at George Washington University in Washington, D.C. He remained there until 1974, when he returned to Charleston and entered into

Fletcher C. Derrick, Jr., M.D.

private practice with Dr. Raymond Rosenblum. In 2006, he decided to semi-retire but still works in the office only, seeing many of his patients of long standing, offering second opinions, and seeing a large group with ED.

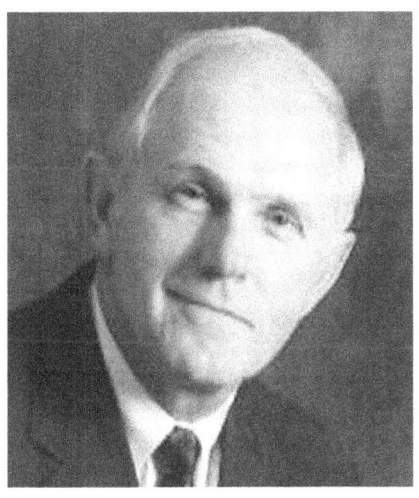

References:

My wife, who taught typing, and is also a writer, aided greatly in editing, and says this booklet can easily be read in about 1½ hours.

Ishak, W.W., MD, FAPA, *The Guidebook of Sexual Medicine*: A and W Publishing Group, Beverly Hill, California, 2008.

INDEX

ForeWord Clarion Review
MEDICAL / SELF-HELP / MALE

Hey Men, Listen Up! How to Get It Up and Keep Getting It Up: A Self Help Book on Erectile Dysfunction

Fletcher C. Derrick Jr., MD
978-1-4392-6475-1
Four Stars (out of Five)

In these harried, post-modern times, when getting accurate answers to straightforward questions sometimes seems impossible, it's a treat to find an easy to read, high quality little book on an awkward subject. Hey Men, Listen Up! is just that book. For men (and the women in their lives) confronted with erection problems, getting fast, informative, and discreet advice without having to slog through the Internet or a highly-technical medical journal is priceless.

Fletcher Derrick has been a practicing urologist for nearly fifty years, and has counseled thousands of men about all aspects of erectile dysfunction. He begins the book with definitions, then a primer on what to expect at what age, and the large role lifestyle choices play in causing or exacerbating erection problems. Stress, alcohol use, weight, hypertension, intimacy barriers, the wrong bike seat and a multitude of other controllable factors are discussed. Derrick suggests a variety of practical tools and changes readers can try at home (or in a hotel room), and how they should proceed if more intervention is needed. Derrick cites statistics and the experiences of his patients when discussing the pharmaceutical, surgical, and over-the-counter options. Each of which are explored with rates of success and possible side effects,.

Certain feminist-minded readers might take issue with the author's depiction of wives (everyone is married, of course, though a stripper makes a cameo appearance).At times, Derrick writes as if a man's spouse is somewhat periphery to sexual function, but then it is a book for men. That said, the friendly, relaxed style he uses is indicative of his exceptional expertise and professional confidence. Middle aged and older men will feel right at home with his humor and well chosen anecdotes from his practice. For example, he writes, "Another patient told me that he and his wife enjoyed sex on Sunday afternoon after church and lunch. He would place a pill in his jacket pocket and when church was over, he would go by the water fountain and take his pill. This was usually about thirty to forty minutes before lunch. When his nose began to get stuffy, he knew the medication was working. Everything worked well in the bedroom as well."

Patty Sutherland

www.ingramcontent.com/pod-product-compliance
Lightning Source LLC
Chambersburg PA
CBHW071305170526
45165CB00003B/1427